Brain Tumor

All you need to know

Dr. Sheila Harrison

Disclaimer

This content serves to provide general information about the disease and aims to empower you to seek prompt medical assistance if necessary to prevent complications. It's essential to stress that this information is not a substitute for consulting a qualified physician. The field of medical science is continually evolving, and due to the dynamic nature of medical knowledge, we recommend seeking expert advice if you encounter any inconsistencies or intend to take action based on the information in this content. Never disregard professional medical guidance or delay treatment based on something you've read online, including this material, or from any other online source. Always remember that the internet cannot cure you; rather, healing comes through the guidance of medical professionals and the providence of God.

Table of contents

Overview

Brain tumors are a diverse and complex group of growths that start within the central nervous system. This includes the brain and spinal cord. Understanding this condition is crucial for several reasons, not only due to their nature but also because of their significant implications for healthcare. This article provides an analysis of brain tumors and explores various aspects of it.

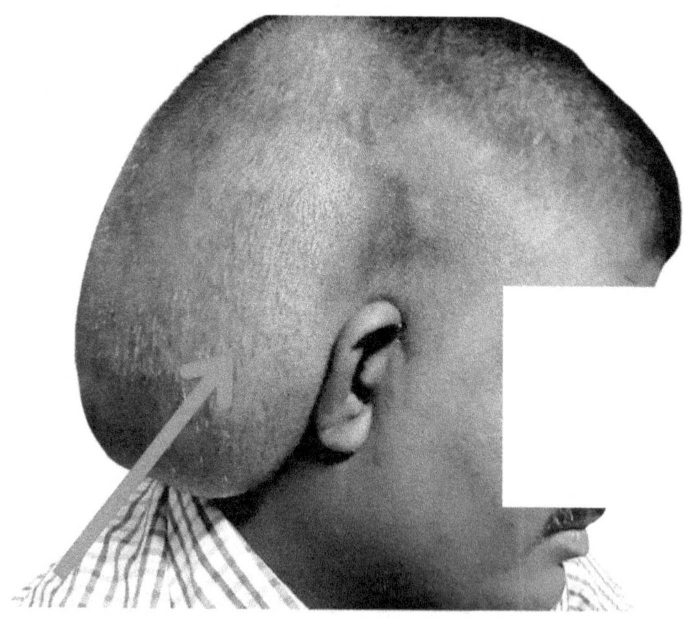

Fully Developed Brain Tumor

Section 1

Types of Brain Tumors

Brain tumors are categorized into two main groups based on their origin and characteristics: primary brain tumors and secondary brain tumors.

Primary brain tumors

Primary brain tumors are those that start within the brain itself. They can be further subdivided into two primary categories based on their behavior:

- **Benign Brain Tumors:** Benign brain tumors are non-cancerous growths. They tend to have well-defined borders and do not invade nearby healthy brain tissue. They typically grow slowly and are less aggressive.

- **Malignant Brain Tumors (Gliomas):** Malignant primary brain tumors, known as gliomas, are cancerous and more aggressive. This category includes various subtypes, each with its unique characteristics:

- ***Glioblastoma Multiforme:*** Glioblastoma is the most aggressive and common form of malignant brain tumor, known for its rapid growth and invasive nature. It carries a poor prognosis.
- ***Anaplastic Astrocytoma:*** Anaplastic astrocytomas are grade III brain tumors with features of malignancy. They grow faster and are more likely to invade nearby brain tissue compared to low-grade gliomas.
- ***Oligodendroglioma:*** They are tumors that arise from oligodendrocytes and are considered grade II or III. They exhibit a characteristic appearance under the microscope.
- ***Ependymoma:*** Ependymomas are tumors that develop from ependymal cells lining the ventricles and the central canal of the spinal cord. They can occur at various locations within the central nervous system.
- ***Medulloblastoma:*** Medulloblastomas are malignant brain tumors that mainly affect children and arise in the cerebellum. They are highly aggressive and require intensive treatment.

- **Other Primary Brain Tumors:** There are various other less common primary brain tumors, each with distinct characteristics, locations as well as behaviors. These tumors may include meningiomas, pituitary adenomas, and schwannomas, among others.

Secondary brain tumors (metastatic brain tumors)

Secondary brain tumors or metastatic brain tumors spread to the brain from cancer originating in other parts of the body. These tumors occur when cancer cells break away from the primary site (e.g., breast, lung, or colon) and travel through the bloodstream or lymphatic system to form tumors within the brain. They often present as multiple lesions and can be challenging to manage due to their diverse origins.

Section 2

Factors Influencing brain tumor size

The size of a brain tumor is influenced by several factors, including:

- **Tumor type:** Different types of brain tumors have varying growth rates and tendencies. Some grow slowly over time, while others can be aggressive and rapidly increase in size.

- **Location:** The location of the tumor within the brain is critical. Tumors situated in critical areas, such as the brainstem or near vital structures, can cause significant issues even when small in size.

- **Individual Variability:** Patient-specific factors, including age, overall health, and genetics, can influence the growth and size of a brain tumor.

- **Early Detection:** Timely diagnosis plays a crucial role in determining the size of a brain tumor. Smaller tumors are often found incidentally during routine imaging for other medical conditions.

Why does the size of the brain tumor matter?

The size of a brain tumor is a key factor in determining its impact on a patient's health and the treatment approach. Smaller tumors are generally associated with a better prognosis and may respond well to less invasive treatment options. In contrast, larger tumors often require more aggressive intervention, and they carry a higher risk of neurological deficits and complications.

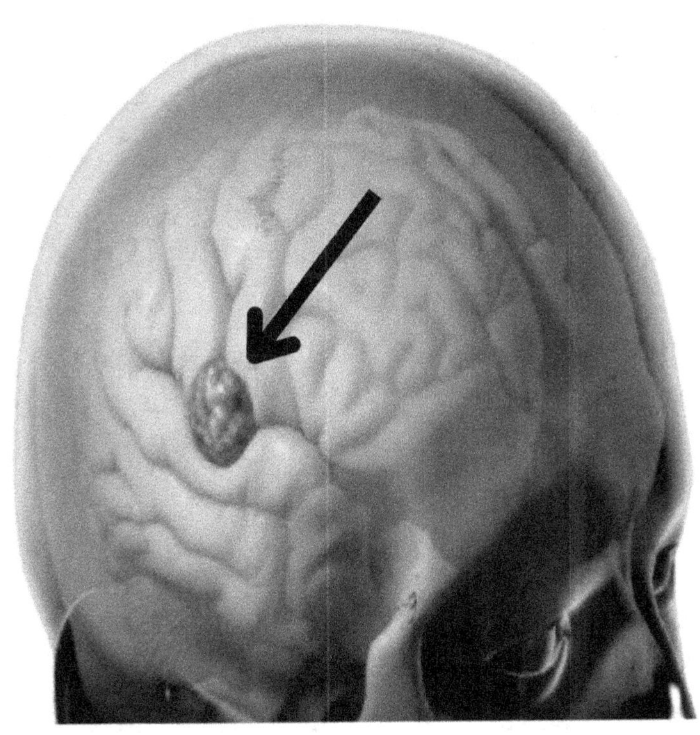

Section 3

Risk factors for brain tumors

A variety of factors influence brain tumors, both primary and secondary, which contribute to their development. Understanding the etiology and risk factors associated with these tumors is essential for assessing potential causes and implementing preventive measures.

Genetic predisposition

Genetic factors are significant in the development of certain types of brain tumors. In some families, there is an increased risk due to inherited genetic mutations. For example, conditions like neurofibromatosis, von Hippel-Lindau disease, and Li-Fraumeni syndrome may have a higher predisposition to brain tumors. Genetic counseling and testing can help identify individuals at risk and guide preventive strategies.

Ionizing radiation exposure

Exposure to ionizing radiation, such as high-dose radiation therapy for the treatment of other cancers or workplace exposure (e.g., nuclear industry workers), is a well-established risk factor. The effects of ionizing radiation on brain tissue can lead to the development of tumors, particularly meningiomas and gliomas. Minimizing unnecessary radiation exposure and following safety guidelines are essential for risk reduction.

Environmental factors

We do not yet fully understand the exact environmental factors contributing to the development of this condition. However, certain environmental factors have been studied for their potential associations. These include exposure to certain chemicals, pesticides, and electromagnetic fields (EMFs). Research into the impact of environmental factors on these tumors is ongoing. We can take precautionary measures, such as limiting exposure to potentially harmful substances and using safety precautions in relevant industries.

- **Viral infections:** Some viral infections have been investigated for their possible links to brain tumors. For example, the

Epstein-Barr virus (EBV) has been associated with certain types of brain lymphomas. However, the relationship between viral infections and tumors is complex and not fully elucidated. Preventive strategies include vaccinations, where available, and general infection control measures.

Family history

Individuals who have family members with brain tumors may have an increased risk of developing brain tumors.

Section 4

Symptoms of brain tumors

Brain tumors often present with a wide array of symptoms. Also, the clinical presentation can vary significantly based on factors such as the tumor's location, size, and rate of growth. The typical clinical symptoms include headaches, seizures, cognitive impairment, sensory and motor changes, behavioral changes, and visual disturbances.

- **Headaches:** Headaches are a frequent symptom of brain tumors. Patients often describe these headaches as persistent, dull, and worsening over time. They can be more intense in the morning, possibly due to increased intracranial pressure when lying down. Headaches due to tumors are different from typical tension or migraine headaches. These should be evaluated by a healthcare professional, especially if they are new or severe.

- **Seizures:** Seizures can be an early sign, particularly in individuals who have never experienced seizures before. The type of seizure can vary, with some individuals experiencing generalized tonic-clonic seizures, while others may have focal seizures that affect specific body parts or functions.

- **Cognitive impairment:** Brain tumors can lead to cognitive changes, such as memory problems, difficulty concentrating, and changes in thinking and reasoning. These cognitive impairments can impact an individual's daily life and are often more pronounced with tumors in areas responsible for cognition.

- **Sensory and motor changes:** Brain tumors located near the brain's sensory or motor regions can lead to changes in sensation as well as motor function. This might manifest as weakness in specific body parts, numbness, tingling, or difficulty coordinating movements.

- **Behavioral changes:** Brain tumors can affect a person's behavior and personality. Individuals may experience alterations in mood, emotions, or behavior, which can be subtle or more pronounced. These changes may be particularly noticeable to family members and close contacts.

- **Visual disturbances:** Tumors that affect the visual pathways or structures within the brain can lead to visual disturbances. These may include blurred or double vision, visual field deficits (partial loss of vision in specific areas), and, in some cases, complete vision loss.

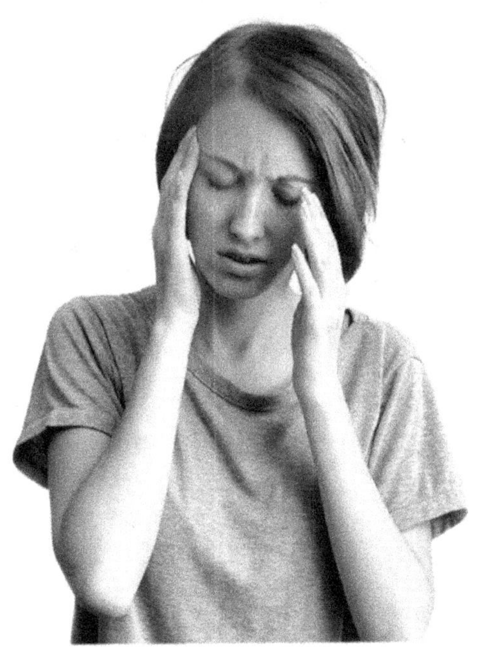

Persistent Headache

Section 5

Brain Tumor Diagnose

Accurate diagnosis of brain tumors is essential for effective treatment planning and improved patient outcomes. Healthcare professionals often use a combination of diagnostic approaches to assess and characterize brain tumors. The choice of diagnostic approaches depends on the individual patient's clinical presentation and the specific characteristics of the suspected brain tumor. Often, a combination of these methods is used to achieve a comprehensive understanding of the tumor, enabling healthcare professionals to make informed treatment decisions tailored to the patient's needs.

Some of the primary diagnostic methods include imaging techniques, biopsy, molecular and genetic testing, and cerebrospinal fluid analysis.

1. Imaging techniques

- **Magnetic Resonance Imaging (MRI):** MRI is a cornerstone of brain tumor diagnosis. It provides detailed, high-resolution images of the brain, allowing healthcare professionals to visualize the tumor's location, size, shape, and proximity to critical structures. Various MRI sequences, such as T1-weighted, T2-weighted, and contrast-enhanced images, offer valuable information about the tumor's characteristics.

- **Computed Tomography (CT):** CT scans use X-rays to create cross-sectional images of the brain. While less detailed than MRI, CT scans are valuable for detecting acute bleeding, and bone involvement, and identifying the presence of a tumor. CT scans are often used when MRI is not feasible or in emergencies.

- **Positron Emission Tomography (PET):** PET scans are used to evaluate the metabolic activity of tumors. By injecting a radioactive tracer into the bloodstream, PET scans can identify areas of the brain with increased glucose metabolism, which is common in rapidly growing tumor cells. PET imaging complements other diagnostic methods to assess tumor aggressiveness.

- **Functional MRI (fMRI):** fMRI is a specialized MRI technique that maps brain activity by measuring changes in blood flow. It helps identify critical brain regions responsible for functions such as speech, motor skills, or sensory perception. fMRI is useful in planning surgery to minimize damage to these areas.

2. Biopsy and histopathological examination

A biopsy involves the surgical removal of a sample of the tumor tissue, which is then examined under a microscope. The histopathological examination provides critical information about the tumor's type, grade, and cellular characteristics. This analysis guides treatment decisions and helps determine the tumor's aggressiveness.

3. Molecular and genetic testing

Advances in molecular and genetic testing have transformed brain tumor diagnosis and treatment. These tests assess specific genetic mutations and molecular markers within the tumor, providing insights into its biological behavior and potential therapeutic targets. Molecular profiling can guide the selection of targeted therapies and precision medicine approaches.

4. Cerebrospinal fluid analysis

Cerebrospinal fluid (CSF) analysis involves the collection and examination of the fluid that surrounds the brain and spinal cord. In some cases, brain tumors can shed cells or release substances into the CSF. Analyzing the CSF can provide valuable information about the tumor's characteristics and help diagnose certain types of the condition, such as leptomeningeal metastases.

Section 6

Brain Tumor Treatment

The management of brain tumors involves a range of treatment strategies. They may be used individually or in combination, depending on their type, location, and stage, as well as the patient's overall health. The choice of treatment strategies is highly individualized and based on a comprehensive assessment of the tumor's characteristics and the patient's overall health. Multidisciplinary teams of healthcare professionals, including neurosurgeons, oncologists, radiologists, and supportive care specialists, collaborate to provide the most effective and patient-centered approach to treatment.

The primary treatment strategies for brain tumors include surgical interventions, radiation therapy, chemotherapy, targeted therapies, immunotherapy, and supportive care.

1. **Surgical interventions**
   - **Craniotomy:** A craniotomy is a surgery in which a healthcare expert temporarily removes a section of the skull to access

and remove the tumor. Doctors commonly use this approach for primary brain tumors when they are accessible and their removal is safe. It allows for tumor biopsy or complete resection.

- **Stereotactic Radiosurgery:** Stereotactic radiosurgery, such as Gamma Knife or CyberKnife, is a non-invasive technique that delivers precisely targeted high-dose radiation to the brain tumor. It is often used for small tumors or for cases where surgical removal may not be suitable due to the tumor's location or the patient's overall health.

- **Endoscopic Surgery:** Endoscopic surgery involves using a small, flexible tube with a camera (endoscope) to access and remove tumors in less invasive ways. It is particularly valuable for tumors in areas that are challenging to reach with traditional surgical approaches.

2. Radiation therapy

- **External Beam Radiation:** External beam radiation therapy involves directing high-energy X-ray beams at the tumor from outside the body. It is often used following surgery to target remaining tumor cells or as a primary treatment for inoperable tumors. Precise planning ensures minimal impact on healthy brain tissue.

- **Brachytherapy:** Brachytherapy involves placing radioactive sources directly inside or very close to the tumor. This technique is used for certain brain tumors, allowing a highly localized, concentrated dose of radiation to be delivered while sparing healthy tissue.

3. Chemotherapy

Chemotherapy involves the administration of drugs, either orally or intravenously, to kill or inhibit the growth of cancer cells. While chemotherapy is not always the primary treatment for brain tumors, it may be used in conjunction with other therapies, particularly for high-grade or recurrent tumors.

4. Targeted therapies

Targeted therapies are drugs designed to specifically target molecular or genetic changes in tumor cells. These therapies can be effective in cases where tumors have specific genetic mutations that make them responsive to targeted treatments.

5. Immunotherapy

Immunotherapy aims to harness the body's immune system to recognize and attack cancer cells. While still in the early stages of development for brain tumors, immunotherapy shows promise, particularly for glioblastoma multiforme and other aggressive brain tumors.

Section 7

Treatment Challenges of Brain Tumors

Brain tumors hold considerable significance within the healthcare landscape for several reasons. These reasons make brain tumors challenging to treat.

- **Complex diagnosis and treatment:** Brain tumors present a complex diagnostic challenge due to their location and the potential for varied symptoms. Accurate diagnosis requires advanced imaging techniques and often invasive procedures like biopsies. Treatment options include surgery, radiation therapy, chemotherapy, and emerging modalities such as immunotherapy.

- **Impact on quality of life:** Brain tumors can severely affect an individual's quality of life. Depending on the tumor's location and type, patients may experience a range of symptoms. These include cognitive impairment, motor deficits, seizures, and personality changes. Managing these symptoms and increasing the patient's well-being is a central concern for healthcare providers.

- **Survival rates and prognosis:** The prognosis for the tumor patients can vary due to factors like tumor type, grade, and patient age. The overall survival rates for malignant brain tumors, particularly glioblastoma multiforme, are often relatively low. This makes early diagnosis and treatment essential.

- **Ongoing research and advancements:** Brain tumor research is an active field, leading to ongoing advancements in diagnostic tools, treatment modalities, and our understanding of the underlying molecular and genetic mechanisms. These advancements offer hope for improved outcomes and potential cures in the future.

Section 8

Prognosis of Brain Tumor Patient

The prognosis for patients with brain tumors can vary widely, influenced by multiple factors. Understanding these factors and their impact on patient outcomes is essential for healthcare providers and patients alike.

Factors influencing prognosis

- **Tumor grade and type:** The grade and type of brain tumor are among the most critical determinants of prognosis. Tumor grade is a measure of how abnormal the tumor cells appear under a microscope and how quickly they are likely to grow and spread. Higher-grade tumors, such as glioblastoma multiforme, are associated with a more aggressive course and poorer prognosis compared to lower-grade tumors. Additionally, the specific tumor type and its location within the brain can significantly affect treatment options and outcomes.

- **Age and general health:** A patient's age and overall health play a significant role in prognosis. Younger individuals generally have better outcomes, as they tend to tolerate aggressive treatments better and may have fewer comorbidities. However, age alone should not be the sole determinant of treatment decisions, as health status, functional independence, and treatment-related side effects should also be considered.

- **Treatment response:** The response to treatment is a critical factor in determining prognosis. Patients who respond well to surgery, radiation therapy, chemotherapy, or targeted therapies may experience more favorable outcomes. Conversely, inadequate treatment responses or tumor progression during therapy can negatively impact prognosis.

Survivorship and quality of life

Survivorship after a brain tumor diagnosis is an essential consideration. Beyond the medical aspects, survivorship encompasses the overall well-being and quality of life for patients and their families. While the journey can be challenging, several factors can contribute to a positive survivorship experience:

- **Rehabilitation and supportive care:** Rehabilitation services, including physical therapy, occupational therapy, and speech therapy, can help patients regain function and improve their quality of life after treatment. Supportive care, including palliative care and pain management, focuses on addressing symptoms and enhancing comfort.

- **Psychosocial support:** Coping with a brain tumor diagnosis and its treatment can be emotionally and psychologically demanding. Access to counseling, support groups, and mental health services can significantly improve the emotional well-being of patients and their families.

- **Long-Term follow-up:** Regular follow-up care is essential for monitoring tumor recurrence or progression. Continued surveillance, including imaging and clinical assessments, helps detect and address any new developments promptly.

- **Patient and caregiver education:** Informed patients and caregivers can actively participate in decision-making and self-care. Education on treatment options, potential side effects as well as strategies for symptom management is critical.

- **Advancements in research:** Ongoing research into the treatment and survivorship is continually improving outcomes and quality of life. Participation in clinical trials and staying informed about the latest developments in brain tumor research can offer hope and opportunities for enhanced treatment approaches.

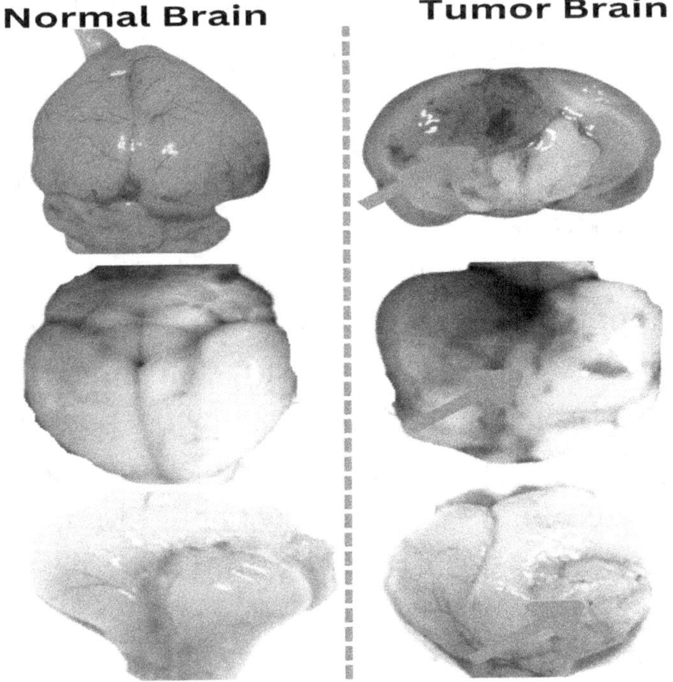

Section 9

Supportive care and symptom management

Recent Advancements in Brain Tumor research

Undoubtedly, brain tumor research is a dynamic and evolving field that has seen significant progress in recent years, offering hope for improved treatments and outcomes. Here, we explore some of the noteworthy recent advancements in this area.

Immunotherapies and checkpoint inhibitors

Immunotherapy has emerged as a promising approach to brain tumor treatment. Checkpoint inhibitors, such as nivolumab and pembrolizumab, have shown potential in enhancing the body's immune response against these tumors, particularly glioblastoma. Clinical trials and research into immunotherapies are ongoing, aiming to improve the efficacy and safety of these treatments.

Precision medicine and personalized treatment

Precision medicine involves tailoring treatments to an individual's unique genetic and molecular profile. In brain tumor research, precision medicine has enabled the identification of specific genetic mutations and molecular markers within tumors. This information guides treatment decisions, allowing for personalized therapies that target the specific characteristics of each patient's tumor.

Innovative surgical techniques

Advances in surgical techniques have improved the precision and safety of tumor removal. Image-guided surgeries, intraoperative MRI, and neuronavigation systems help surgeons locate and remove tumors with greater accuracy while minimizing damage to healthy brain tissue. Minimally invasive approaches, including endoscopic surgery, reduce post-operative complications and recovery times.

Blood-brain barrier disruption for drug delivery

The blood-brain barrier (BBB) is a protective barrier that can impede the delivery of therapeutic drugs to brain tumors. Researchers have made further progress in developing methods to temporarily disrupt the BBB, allowing for more effective drug delivery. This approach has the potential to enhance the effectiveness of chemotherapy and targeted therapies.

Novel targeted therapies and clinical trials

The discovery of new molecular targets and pathways within brain tumors has led to the development of novel targeted therapies. These drugs are designed to block specific tumor-promoting mechanisms. Additionally, an increasing number of clinical trials are testing innovative treatments and therapies for brain tumors, providing patients with access to the latest advancements in care.

These recent advances in brain tumor research reflect the dedication of researchers and healthcare professionals to improve the understanding and treatment of these complex and often challenging diseases. As research continues further to expand our knowledge of brain tumors and their molecular intricacies, there is hope for more effective treatments, increased survival rates, and improved quality of life for patients affected by these conditions.

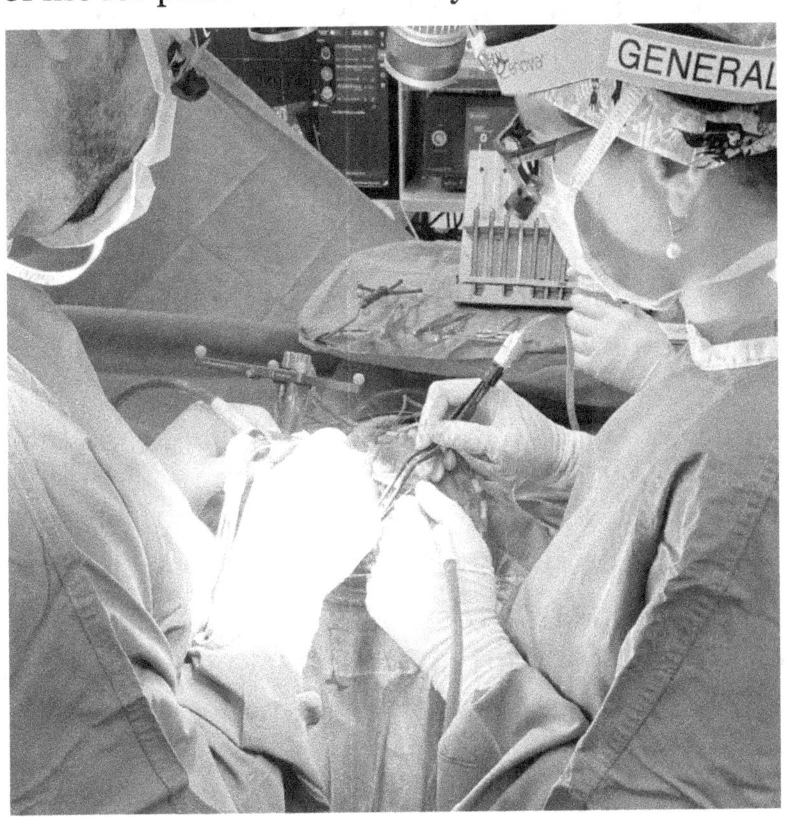

Section 10

FAQ on Brain Tumor

Are high cholesterol and brain tumors related?

Not exactly. High cholesterol and brain tumors are not directly linked. While they share some risk factors, such as lifestyle choices, high cholesterol primarily affects cardiovascular health. However, it can indirectly impact brain health by affecting blood flow and inflammation, though it does not directly cause brain tumors.

Can a brain tumor be a sign of weak bones?

No. A brain tumor is not typically a sign of weak bones. These two conditions are generally unrelated. Certain cancers that spread to the bones can weaken the bones. However, a primary brain tumor is not directly linked to bone health.

Can brain tumors affect existing kidney diseases?

It may. Brain tumors typically do not directly affect existing kidney diseases. However, interactions between treatments, fluid balance, electrolyte imbalances, compromised immune systems, stress, and overall health require careful management in patients with both conditions. Coordination among healthcare specialists is crucial for effective care.

Can brain tumors affect liver diseases?

It may. Brain tumors do not typically directly affect liver diseases. However, the treatments, medications, and overall health management for both conditions can interact and potentially impact each other. Coordination between healthcare providers is essential for individuals dealing with both a brain tumor and liver disease to ensure the best care and minimize potential complications.

Can brain tumors cause heart problems?

It may. Brain tumors can indirectly lead to heart problems by affecting the central nervous system and increasing intracranial pressure, which influences heart rate and blood pressure. Seizures, medication side effects, stress, and physical limitations may also contribute to heart-related issues in some cases. Coordination between specialists is crucial for comprehensive care when dealing with both conditions.

Can CT scans detect brain tumors?

CT scan is an imaging technique that has proven to be highly useful in diagnosing a wide range of medical conditions, including brain tumors. It is a quick and relatively non-invasive procedure, making it a preferred choice for many patients and healthcare professionals. However, while CT scans are powerful tools, they do have some limitations when it comes to detecting brain tumors. These limitations become evident when considering the size, location, and type of tumor. In this article, we will explore the capabilities and limitations of CT scans in diagnosing brain tumors.

What is the capability of a CT Scan in identifying brain tumors?

Among the various diagnostic tools available, the CT (computed tomography) scan is a widely used imaging technique for brain tumors. CT scans or computed axial tomography scans (CAT scans), are a type of medical imaging. These scans use X-rays to create cross-sectional images of the body.

Brain tumors, on the other hand, are abnormal growths of cells within the brain. They can be either benign (non-cancerous) or malignant (cancerous). They may originate within the brain (primary) or spread to the brain from other parts of the body (secondary). Early detection is crucial for effective treatment and improved outcomes, making diagnostic tools like CT scans quite useful.

What factors can affect the efficacy of CT Scans in detecting brain tumors?

There are various factors on which the efficacy of CT Scans depends in detecting brain tumors. Some of them are:

Size of the tumor

One of the crucial factors in the effectiveness of CT scans in detecting brain tumors is the size of the tumor. Small tumors may not always be visible on a CT scan, especially if they are located deep within the brain. Larger tumors are more likely to be detected, as they cause structural changes in the brain. This is a limitation to consider, as early detection of brain tumors can significantly impact treatment options and patient outcomes.

Tumor type and location

CT scans are excellent at identifying the presence of tumors in the brain. However, they may not always provide a definitive diagnosis regarding the type of tumor. Distinguishing between different types of brain tumors, such as gliomas, meningiomas, or metastatic tumors, often requires additional imaging or diagnostic tests, such as MRI (magnetic resonance imaging) or a biopsy. Additionally, the location of the tumor within the brain can affect its visibility on a CT scan. Tumors located near bone or areas with high-density structures can be challenging to detect with CT alone.

Radiation exposure

While CT scans are valuable tools, they involve exposure to ionizing radiation. Repeated CT scans over a short period can pose health risks, especially to sensitive populations such as children and pregnant women. In cases where there is a need for continuous monitoring, MRI, which does not use ionizing radiation, may be a safer alternative.

Combining imaging techniques

In many cases, healthcare professionals use a combination of imaging techniques to provide a more comprehensive evaluation of brain tumors. For instance, MRI is excellent for capturing detailed images of soft tissues, and it is often employed alongside CT scans. This multi-modal approach can help in precise tumor localization, characterization, and treatment planning.

In conclusion, CT scans can indeed play a vital role in the detection of brain tumors. They are efficient in identifying the presence of tumors and are invaluable in emergency situations to quickly assess potentially life-threatening conditions. However, the efficacy of CT scans depends on various factors, including tumor size, type, and location. To obtain a comprehensive diagnosis and treatment plan, it is common for healthcare providers to combine CT scans with other imaging techniques such as MRI or perform additional tests like biopsies. Ultimately, the early detection and accurate diagnosis of brain tumors are crucial for providing patients with the best possible care and improving their chances of successful treatment and recovery. Patients with concerns about brain tumors should consult with their healthcare providers to determine the most appropriate diagnostic approach for their specific case.

What is the normal size of a brain tumor?

Brain tumors can be a frightening diagnosis, with the potential to disrupt one's life and health. When it comes to brain tumors, size matters, as it can have a significant impact on prognosis, symptoms, and treatment options. In this article, we will delve into the concept of a normal size for a brain tumor, exploring the key factors that influence it and the implications for patients.

How are brain tumor sizes classified?

The brain tumor sizes can be classified based on size using TNM classification of malignant tumors. The T-staging system can differentiate the tumors based on their size. T1 Brain Tumors represent the smallest category, measuring 2 centimeters or less in their greatest dimension. T2 Brain Tumors are of moderate size, exceeding 2 centimeters but not surpassing 4 centimeters. T3 Brain Tumors are notably larger and may exhibit signs of invading critical regions within the brain. These tumors are comparable to T4 head and neck tumors, which can encroach upon structures like the carotid artery. T4 Brain Tumors, analogous to their head and neck counterparts, are the most advanced and concerning, with the potential to infiltrate essential brain structures. This adapted T-staging system serves as a valuable tool for comprehending the extent of brain tumors, aiding in diagnosis, treatment planning, and effective communication among healthcare professionals.

www.ingramcontent.com/pod-product-compliance
Lightning Source LLC
Chambersburg PA
CBHW070748260726
48660CB00007B/3022